BREAD MACHINE COOKBOOK 2021

Ultimate Cookbook To Try Tasty Quick And Easy Homemade Recipes With Your Bread Machine

By
Caren Cooper

Copyright © 2021

All rights reserved. No part of this publication may be reproduced or distributed in any form or by any means, electronic or mechanical, photocopying, scanning, recording or otherwise, without prior written permission from the publisher and the author.

Disclaimer of Warranty / Limit of Liability: The author and the publisher are not a licensed physician, medical professional or practitioner and offers no medical counseling, treatments or diagnoses. The author and the publisher make no warranties with respect to the accuracy and completeness of the contents of this work. All the nutritional facts contained in this book is provided for informational purposes only. The information is based on the specific ingredients, measurements and brands used to make the recipe. Therefore, the nutritional facts in this work in no way is intended to be a guarantee of the actual nutritional value of the recipe made by the reader. The author and the publisher will not be responsible for any damages resulting in reliance of the reader on the nutritional information.

The content presented herein, has not been evaluated by the U.S. Food and Drug Administration, and it is not intended to cure or diagnose any disease. This book isn't intended as a substitute for medical advice as physicians. Full medical clearance from a licensed physician should be obtained before beginning any diet. The advice and strategies contained herein may not be suitable for every situation. Neither the author nor the publisher claims no responsibility to any person or entity for any liability, damage or loss caused directly or indirectly as a result of the use, application or interpretation of the information presented in this work.

The publisher publishes its books in a variety of print and electronic formats. Some content that appears in print may not be available in electronic, and vice versa.

Table Of Contents

INTRODUCTION 8

CHAPTER 1: HOW TO BAKE USING A BREAD MACHINE 12

CHAPTER 2: HOW TO USE A BREAD MACHINE 16
    Meet Your New Bread Machine 16
    Main Ingredients 17

CHAPTER 3: WHAT ARE THE MOST COMMON INGREDIENTS 22

CHAPTER 4: TIPS AND TRICKS IN ORDER TO HAVE A BETTER FINAL PRODUCT AND TO SAVE MONEY AND TIME 26

CHAPTER 5: PERFECT FOR BREAKFAST 32
    1.   Breakfast Bread 32

CHAPTER 6: WHOLE-WHEAT BREAD 34
    2.   Whole Wheat Bread 34

CHAPTER 7: CLASSIC BREAD 36
    3.   Almond Flour Bread 36

CHAPTER 8: SPICE AND HERB BREAD 38
    4.   Herb Bread 38

CHAPTER 9: SOURDOUGH BREAD 40
    5.   Garlic and Herb Flatbread Sourdough 40

CHAPTER 10: SWEET BREAD 42
    6. Brownie Bread 42
    7.   Black Forest Bread 44

CHAPTER 11: CHEESE BREAD 46
    8.   Parmesan Tomato Basil Bread 46
    9.   Cheese Buttermilk Bread 48

CHAPTER 12: DOUGH RECIPES 50
    10. Cheddar Biscuits 50

CHAPTER 13: BUNS & BREAD 52
11. BUNS WITH COTTAGE CHEESE 52

CHAPTER 14: BREAD MACHINE RECIPES 54
12. GREAT PLUM BREAD 54
13. LIME BREAD 56

CHAPTER 15: NUT AND SEED BREAD 58
14. FLAX AND SUNFLOWER SEED BREAD 58
15. HONEY AND FLAXSEED BREAD 60

CHAPTER 16: VEGETABLE BREAD 62
16. BANANA-LEMON LOAF 62
17. ORANGE DATE BREAD 64

CHAPTER 17: BASIC BREAD 66
18. GLUTEN-FREE BREAD 66

CHAPTER 18: PLEASURE BREAD 68
19. CRISP WHITE BREAD 68

CHAPTER 19: CAKES AND QUICK BREAD 70
20. HONEY POUND CAKE 70

CHAPTER 20: MEAT BREAD 72
21. FRENCH HAM BREAD 72

CHAPTER 21: MULTI-GRAIN BREAD 74
22. FRENCH CRUSTY LOAF BREAD 74

CHAPTER 22: HOLIDAY BREAD 76
23. PUMPKIN BREAD 76

CHAPTER 23: KETO BREAD RECIPES 78
24. SIMPLE MILK BREAD 78
25. TOAST BREAD 80
26. WALNUT BREAD 81

CHAPTER 24: INTERNATIONAL BREAD 84
27. GERMAN PUMPERNICKEL BREAD 84

CHAPTER 25: FRUIT AND VEGETABLE BREAD 86
28. Banana Bread 86
29. Orange and Walnut Bread 88

CHAPTER 26: WHITE BREAD 90
30. Basic White Bread 90

CHAPTER 27: SPECIAL BREAD RECIPES 92
31. Gluten-Free Simple Sandwich Bread 92
32. Grain-Free Chia Bread 94

CHAPTER 28: ROLLS AND PIZZA 96
33. Sweet Potato Rolls 96

CHAPTER 29: ITALIAN STYLED 98
34. Fruit Bread 98
35. Marzipan Cherry Bread 100
36. Ginger Prune Bread 102

CHAPTER 30: FAMOUS BREAD RECIPES 104
37. Bread Machine Glazed Yeast Doughnuts 104
38. Bread Machine Kalamata Olive Bread 107
39. Dark Pumpernickel Bread 109
40. Bread Machine Hamburger Buns 111

CONCLUSION 114

CONVERSION TABLES 116
Measuring Equivalent Chart 116
Gluten-Free – Conversion Tables 118
Flour: Quantity and Weight 119
Sugar: Quantity and Weight 119
Cream: Quantity and Weight 120
Butter: Quantity and Weight 120
Oven Temperature Equivalent Chart 121

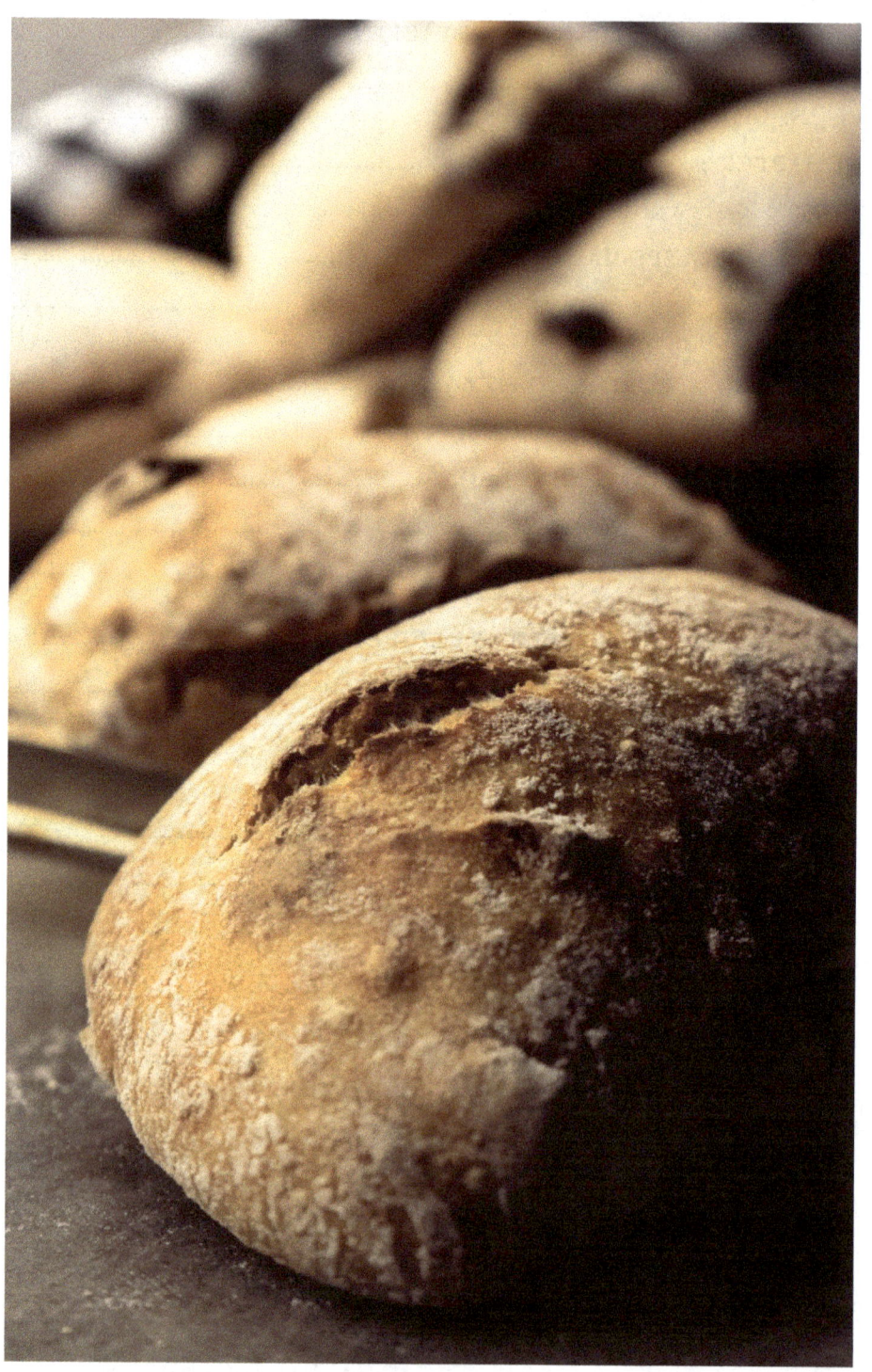

Introduction

Bread making machine, otherwise known as a bread maker, is a home-based appliance that transforms uncooked ingredients into bread. It is made up of a saucepan for bread (or "tin"), with one or more built-in paddles at the bottom, present in the center of a small special-purpose oven. This little oven is usually operated via a control panel via a simple in-built computer utilizing the input settings. Some bread machines have diverse cycles for various forms of dough — together with white bread, whole grain, European-style (occasionally called "French"), and dough-only (for pizza dough and formed loaves baked in a traditional oven). Many also have a timer to enable the bread machine to work without the operator's attendance, and some high-end models allow the user to program a customized period.

To bake bread, ingredients are measured in a specified order into the bread pan (usually first liquids, with solid ingredients layered on top), and then the pan is put in the bread maker. The order of ingredients is important because contact with water triggers the instant yeast used in bread makers, so the yeast and water have to be kept separate until the program starts.

It takes the machine several hours to make a bread loaf. The products are rested first and brought to an optimal temperature. Stir with a paddle, and the ingredients are then shaped into flour. Use optimal temperature regulation, and the dough is then confirmed and then cooked.

When the bread has been baked, the bread maker removes the pan. Then leaving a slight indentation from the rod to which the paddle is connected. The finished loaf's shape is often regarded as unique. Many initial bread machines manufacture a vertically slanted towards, square, or cylindrical loaf that is significantly dissimilar from commercial bread; however, more recent units typically have a more conventional horizontal pan. Some bread machines use two paddles to form two lb. loaf in regular rectangle shape.

Bread machine recipes are often much smaller than regular bread recipes. Sometimes standardized based on the machine's pan capacity, most popular in the US market is 1.5 lb. /700 g units. Most recipes are written for that capacity; however, two lb. /900 g units are not uncommon. There are prepared bread mixes, specially made for bread makers, containing pre-measured ingredients and flour and yeast, flavorings, and sometimes dough conditioners.

Bread makers are also fitted with a timer for testing when bread-making starts. For example, this allows them to be loaded at night but only begin baking in the morning to produce a freshly baked bread for breakfast. They may also be set only for making dough, for example, for making pizza. Apart from bread, some can also be set to make other things like jam, pasta dough, and Japanese rice cake. Some of the new developments in the facility of the machine includes automatically adding nut. It also contains fruit from a tray during the kneading process. Bread makers typically take between three and four hours to bake a loaf. However, recent "quick bake" modes have become standard additions, many of which can produce a loaf in less than an hour.

CHAPTER 1:

How to Bake Using a Bread Machine

Home bread makers are designed in such a way that any housewife can use it without much difficulty. However, for the stove to serve for a long time, and the bread always turns out to be high, lush, and tasty, specific rules must be followed.

You need to install the bread maker away from batteries, stoves, and sunlight since all temperature factors affect the oven's heating.

Before each new cooking, make sure that no crumbs are stuck on the blades and that the edge is on the shaft until it stops.

When laying the components, you must strictly follow the instructions: for example, if you want to start with liquids, then first pour in water, milk, or other liquid product. The flour is run to cover the liquid layer entirely, and then different dry ingredients are poured. Salt, sugar, hard butter (butter) is placed in the grooves made in the stacked layers to not come into contact with each other. Then, in the middle of the dry components layer, depression is caused, and yeast is poured into it (the depression should not reach the liquid coating).

A container with food is placed in the oven (usually there are special fasteners), the lid is closed, and the oven is plugged into a power outlet. Choose a program, the finished product's size, and the crust (if provided in the model). Press the "Start" or "Start" button. After that, the kneading process begins. If the oven has a timer, then you can set the time for preparing the bread for a specific time.

During kneading, the dough is checked by periodically opening the lid. To make good bread, the dough should be slightly sticky to the touch. If the dough is too soft and moist, add a little flour; if it turns out to be very dense, add liquid.

It is essential to assess the state of the dough during the lifting process. The dough may rise too high on hot days, and then it falls out of the mold and falls on the heating coils.

To not change the baking program, the dough can be punctured in several places to fall off. Or, cancel the originally specified program and set the mode, which in many models is called "Baking only."

All additives fall asleep after the stove signal about the end of the kneading, also, by a timer indicating that the kneading process is completed. If the stove has an automatic addition mode, then all components are poured into a special compartment at the beginning of cooking, as we have already mentioned earlier.

At the end of the cycle, the bread maker beeps. It either turns off itself in automatic mode, or you should press the "Stop" button. After that, the lid is opened, gloves are put on. The bread is then taken out (it is not recommended to lean close to the open stove and also rely on it).

Then turn the mold over the board, take out the bread, put it on the wire rack so that it cools down gradually. They then turn off the stove from the network and let it cool down (it is not recommended to start preparing a new portion of bread without waiting for the furnace to cool down).

It is recommended to use freshly baked bread for food within two to three days. It must be remembered that products containing eggs stale faster. Bread containing honey and butter retains its freshness and elasticity longer.

CHAPTER 2:

How to Use a Bread Machine

Meet Your New Bread Machine

Hot golden crescents, freshly baked breakfast cakes, aromatic tea cakes and delicious cakes to accompany your morning coffee All of these can be cooked with a bread machine in minutes and with a little effort on your part. Also, these delicious and healthy baked goods can be made with the simplest and most common ingredients. The only special thing you need to add is your love and creativity! As for the boring and routine tasks, such as baking, mixing, stirring, the bread machine will take care of them leaving you the best and most enjoyable, that is, the choice of the recipe and the choice of ingredients. Isn't this a great way to enjoy the unique aroma and flavor of exactly the type of baked goods you need?

Even if you're not good at using modern appliances, put your worries behind you, because bread machines have simple, easy-to-use controls. They are fun and easy to use! Besides making fresh bread, they can also make and knead any type of dough, bake dough out of the box, and even make dough jam. When you get to know this handy device, it will truly become an essential and exceptional aid in your kitchen.

It's so simple

Insert the baking sheet into the machine.

Attach the dough blades.

Add ingredients as shown in your machine manual.

Close the lid.

Turn on the machine.

Select the required function.

What Else Can It Do?

Different bread machines may differ in their design, capacity, number of accessories, and programs available. When choosing your bread machine, think of your own preferences and needs: What will you do with the machine? Do you need any particular programs and additional modes, or is the basic functionality enough?

Bread machines can knead the dough, let it rest, bake a crunchy baguette, make sweet cupcakes or unleavened bread, and much more.

Main Ingredients

The ingredients needed for bread making are very simple: flour, yeast, salt, and liquid. There are other ingredients that add flavor, texture, and nutrition to your bread, such as sugar, fats, and eggs. The basic ingredients include:

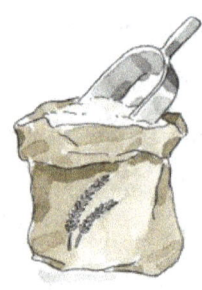

Flour is the foundation of bread.

The protein and gluten in flour forms a network that traps the carbon dioxide and alcohol produced by the yeast. Flour also provides simple sugar to feed the yeast and it provides flavor, depending on the type of flour used in the recipe.

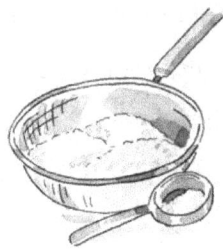

Yeast is a living organism that increases when the right amount of moisture, food, and heat are applied. Rapidly multiplying yeast gives off carbon dioxide and ethyl alcohol.

When yeast is allowed to go through its life cycle completely, the finished bread is more flavorful.

The best yeast for bread machines is bread machine yeast or active dry yeast, depending on your bread machine model.

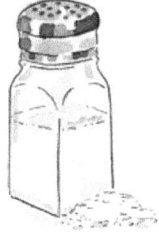

Salt strengthens gluten and slows the rise of the bread by retarding the action of the yeast. A slower rise allows the flavors of the bread to develop better, and it will be less likely the bread will rise too much.

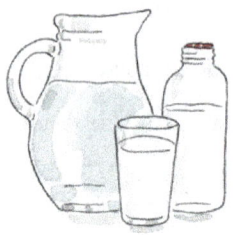

Liquid activates the yeast and dissolves the other ingredients. The most commonly used liquid is water, but ingredients such as milk can also be substituted. Bread made with water will have a crisper crust, but milk produces rich, tender bread that offers more nutrition and browns easier.

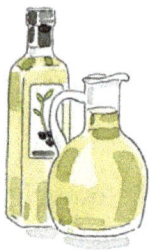

Oils and fats add flavor, create a tender texture, and help brown the crust. Bread made with fat stays fresh longer because moisture loss in the bread is slowed. This component can also inhibit gluten formation, so the bread does not rise as high.

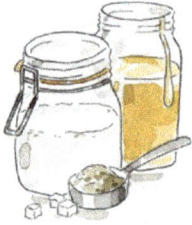

Sugar is the source of food for the yeast. It also adds sweetness, tenderness, and color to the crust. Too much sugar can inhibit gluten growth or cause the dough to rise too much and collapse. Other sweeteners can replace sugar, such as honey, molasses, maple syrup, brown sugar, and corn syrup.

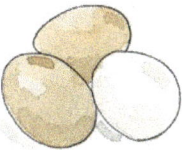

Eggs add protein, flavor, color, and a tender crust. Eggs contain an emulsifier, lecithin, which helps create a consistent texture, and a leavening agent, which helps the bread rise well.

CHAPTER 3:

What are the Most Common Ingredients

Bread making consists of a few very basic ingredients flour, liquids, yeast, butter, etc. Knowing the role of these ingredients helps you to understand the baking process. Moreover, the order in which you add ingredients is crucial when making bread in your bread machine. Do not commit the cardinal sin of bread making by adding the ingredients randomly to the bread pan. The following sections highlight the correct order to put ingredients in the bread pan to bake perfect loaves of bread.

Water/Milk

All of the other basic bread ingredients, including flour, salt, and yeast, need a liquid medium to do their respective tasks. Water is the most common liquid ingredient; milk, buttermilk, cream, and juice are some common substitutes.

The liquid is usually the first ingredient to be added to the bread pan. This is very important as it maintains the ideal texture of your bread. The liquid should not be cold; ensure that it is lukewarm (between 80 and 90°F) whenever possible.

Butter/Oil

Butter, oil, or fat is usually added after the liquid. This is what gives bread crust its attractive brown color and crispy texture. Do not use cold butter that has just been taken out of the refrigerator. You can either microwave it for a few seconds or keep it at room temperature until it gets soft.

Sugar/honey (if using)

Sweet ingredients such as honey, corn syrup, maple syrup, and sugar are usually added after the butter as they mix easily with water and butter. However, the sweetener can be added before the butter as well. Sugar, honey, etc. serve as a feeding medium for yeast, so fermentation is stronger with the addition of sweet ingredients.

Eggs (if using)

Eggs need to be at room temperature before they are added to the bread pan. If the eggs are taken from the refrigerator, keep them outside at room temperature until they are no longer cold. They keep the crust tender and add protein and flavor to the bread.

Chilled Ingredients

If you are using any other ingredient that is kept chilled, such as cheese, milk, buttermilk or cream, keep it outside at room temperature until it is no longer cold, or microwave it for a few seconds to warm it up.

Salt

Use table salt or non-iodized salt for better results. Salt that is high in iodine can hamper the activity of the yeast and create problems with fermentation.

Furthermore, salt itself is a yeast inhibitor and should not be touching yeast directly; that is why salt and yeast are never added together or one after another.

Spices (if using)

Spices such as cinnamon, nutmeg, and ginger are often used to add flavor to the bread. They may be added before or after the flour.

Flour

Flour is the primary ingredient for any bread recipe. It contains gluten (except for the gluten-free flours) and protein, and when the yeast produces alcohol and carbon dioxide, the gluten and protein trap the alcohol and carbon dioxide to initiate the bread-making process.

There are many different types of flours used for preparing different types of bread. Bread machine flour or white bread flour is the most common type as it is suitable for most bread recipes.

It's so versatile because it contains an ideal proportion of protein for bread baking.

Usually, flour is stored at room temperature, but if you keep your flour in your fridge, allow it to warm up before using it.

Seeds (if using)

If a recipe calls for adding seeds such as sunflower seeds or caraway seeds, these should be added after the flour. However, when two different flours are being used, it is best to add the seeds in between the flours for a better mix.

Yeast

Yeast is the ingredient responsible for initiating the vital bread-making process of fermentation. Yeast needs the right amount of heat, moisture and liquid to grow and multiply. When yeast multiplies, it releases alcohol and carbon dioxide.

You can use active dry yeast or bread machine yeast (both will be available in local grocery stores). Cool, dry places are ideal to store yeast packs.

Yeast is added to the bread pan last, after the flour and other dry ingredients. (For certain types of bread, like fruit and nut bread, yeast is technically not the last ingredient, as the fruits or nuts are added later by the machine. However, yeast is the last ingredient to be added before starting the bread machine.)

CHAPTER 4:

Tips and tricks in Order to have a Better Final Product and to Save Money and Time

When you are using a bread machine for the first time, it's common to have some concerns. However, they are quite easy to fix.

The following are some useful tips and quick-and-easy fixes for the most common problems encountered while baking bread in a bread machine.

Dough Check

You can check the progress of the dough while the bread machine is mixing the ingredients. Take a quick check after 5 minutes of kneading. An ideal dough with the right amount of dry and wet ingredients makes one smooth ball and feels slightly tacky.

You can open the lid to evaluate the dough. Do not worry about interfering with the kneading process by opening the lid; the bread structure won't be affected even if you poke it to get a feel for the dough.

If the dough feels too wet/moist or does not form into a ball shape, you can add 1 tablespoon of flour at a time and check again after a few minutes. If you feel that the dough is too dry, or it has formed two or three small balls, you can add 1 teaspoon of water at a time and check again after a few minutes.

Fruit/Nut Bread

When making fruit or nut bread, it is very important to add fruits or nuts at the right time. Not all bread machines come with a nut/fruit dispenser or hopper. If yours doesn't have one, don't worry; the machine will signal you with a beep series when it's time to add the fruits or nuts.

Citrus Ingredients

Citrus ingredients such as lemon zest, orange zest, orange juice, lemon juice, and pineapple juice can create issues with yeast fermentation if added in excess. Do not add more than the quantity specified in a recipe. The same goes for alcohol and cinnamon.

Salt Adjustment

When making small loaves (around 1 pound), sometimes the loaf rises more or less than expected. In many such instances, the issue is with the quantity of salt added. To avoid problems, try using less salt or cutting back on the quantity specified in the recipe. Using sea salt or coarse salt can also help prevent problems with small loaves.

Bread Collapse

The amount of yeast is very important for proper rising. The most common reason for bread collapse during the baking process is adding too much or too little yeast. Do not add more yeast than specified in the recipe. Also, check the expiration date on the yeast pack; freshly packed yeast provides the best results. Other reasons for bread collapse are using cold water and adding excess salt.

Failure to Rise

Many factors can contribute to the failure of dough to rise completely. Insufficient gluten content, miscalculated ingredients, excess salt, excess sugar, and using cold ingredients are the most common reasons. Always warm any chilled ingredients or place them at room temperature for a while before adding them to the bread pan. However, if you are warming any ingredients in your oven, make sure not to overheat them. They need to be lukewarm, at between 80 and 90°F, and not too hot. Also make sure that the yeast does not come in direct contact with the salt, as this creates problems with rising (that is why yeast is added last).

Texture Troubles

- If your bread has a coarse texture, try adding more salt and reducing the amount of liquid.
- If your bread looks small and feels dense, try using flour with higher protein content. Bread flour has a sufficient amount of protein, but slightly denser loaves are common when you use heavier flours such as rye flour and whole wheat flour. Use additional ingredients such as fruits, nuts, and vegetables in their specified quantities. Adding too

much of such ingredients will make your loaf too heavy, small, and dense.

- Moist or gummy loaves are less common, but it can happen if you have added too much liquid or used too much sugar. Too much liquid can also result in a doughy center.

- If your bread has an unbrowned top, try adding more sugar. This can also happen if your bread machine has a glass top.

- If your loaf has a mushroom top, it is probably due to too much yeast or water. Try reducing the amount of water and/or yeast.

- Sometimes a baked loaf has some flour on one side. When you bake the next time, try to remove any visible flour during the kneading cycle with a rubber spatula.

- If your loaf has an overly dark crust, try using the Medium crust setting next time. This also happens if you've added too much sugar and when you fail to take out the bread pan after the end of the baking process. It is always advisable to remove the bread pan right after the process is complete.

- If your loaf has a sunken top, it is probably because of using too much liquid or overly hot ingredients. This is also common during humid or warm weather.

Excess Rise

Many times, a loaf rises more than expected; the most common reasons are too much yeast, too little salt, and using cold water. But also make sure that the capacity of your bread pan is sufficient for the size of loaf you have selected; trying to make a large loaf in a small bread pan will obviously lead to such trouble.

Paddles

After the bread machine completes its baking process the paddles may remain inside the bread loaf. Allow the freshly made bread to cool down and then place it on a cutting board and gently take out the paddles.

Spraying the paddles with a cooking spray before you add the ingredients to the bread pan will make it easier to clean them after the bread is baked.

Cleaning

After you take the baked loaf from the bread pan, do not immerse the pan in water. Rather, fill it with warm soapy water.

CHAPTER 5:

Perfect for Breakfast

1. Breakfast Bread

Preparation Time: 15 minutes

Cooking Time: 40 minutes

Servings: 16 slices

Ingredients:

- ½ tsp. Xanthan gum
- ½ tsp. salt
- 2 Tbsp. coconut oil
- ½ cup butter, melted
- 1 tsp. baking powder
- 2 cups of almond flour
- Seven eggs

Directions:

1. Preheat the oven to 355F.
2. Beat eggs in a bowl on high for 2 minutes.
3. Add coconut oil and butter to the eggs and continue to beat.

4. Line a pan with baking paper and then pour the beaten eggs.
5. Pour in the rest of the ingredients and mix until it becomes thick.
6. Bake until a toothpick comes out dry. It takes 40 to 45 minutes.

Nutrition:

Calories: 234

Fat: 23g

Carb: 1g

Protein: 7g

CHAPTER 6:

Whole-Wheat Bread

2. Whole Wheat Bread

Preparation Time: 9 Minutes

Cooking Time: 4 Hours

Servings: 12 slices

Ingredients:

- Lukewarm water
- Olive oil
- Whole wheat flour sifted
- Salt
- Soft brown sugar
- Dried milk powder, skimmed
- Fast-acting, easy-blend dried yeast

Directions:

1. Add the water and olive oil to your machine, followed by half of the flour.

2. Now apply the salt, sugar, dried milk powder, and remaining flour.
3. Make a little well or dip at the top of the flour. Then carefully place the yeast into it, making sure it doesn't come into contact with any liquid.
4. Set the wholemeal or whole-wheat setting according to your machine's manual, and alter the crust setting to your particular liking.
5. Once baked, carefully remove the bowl from the machine and remove the loaf, placing it on a wire rack to cool. I prefer not to add any toppings to this particular loaf, but you can, of course, experiment and add whatever you want.
6. Once cool, remove the paddle; and, for the very best results, slice with a serrated bread knife. Enjoy!

Nutrition:

Calories: 160

Carbs: 30.1g

Fat: 3,1g

Protein: 5g

CHAPTER 7:

Classic Bread

3. Almond Flour Bread

Preparation Time: 10 Minutes
Cooking Time: 10 Minutes
Servings: 10

Ingredients:

- Four egg whites
- Two egg yolks
- 2 cups almond flour
- 1/4 cup butter, melted
- 2 tbsp. psyllium husk powder
- 1 1/2 tbsp. baking powder
- 1/2 tsp. xanthan gum
- Salt
- 1/2 cup + 2 tbsp. warm water
- 2 1/4 tsp. yeast

Directions:

1. Make use of a small mixing bowl to combine the dry ingredients except for the yeast.
2. In the bread machine pan, add all the wet ingredients.
3. Add all of your dry ingredients from the lower mixing bowl to the bread machine pan. Top with the yeast.
4. Set the bread machine to the basic bread setting.
5. When the bread is completed, remove the bread machine pan from the bread machine.
6. Let cool a little before moving to a cooling rack.
7. The bread can be stored for up to 4 days on the counter and three months in the freezer.

Nutrition:

Calories: 110

Carbohydrates: 2.4g

Protein: 4g

Fat: 10g

CHAPTER 8:

Spice and Herb Bread

4. Herb Bread

Preparation Time: 1 hour 20 minutes

Cooking Time: 50 minutes (20+30 minutes)

Servings: 1 loaf

Ingredients:

- 3/4 to 7/8 cup milk
- 1 tablespoon Sugar
- 1 teaspoon Salt
- tablespoon Butter or margarine
- 1/3 cup chopped onion
- cups bread flour
- 1/2 teaspoon Dried dill
- 1/2 teaspoon Dried basil
- 1/2 teaspoon Dried rosemary
- 11/2 teaspoon Active dry yeast

Directions:

1. Place all the Ingredients in the bread pan. Select medium crus then the rapid bake cycle. Press starts.
2. After 5-10 minutes, observe the dough as it kneads, if you hear straining sounds in your machine or if the dough appears stiff and dry, add 1 tablespoon Liquid at a time until the dough becomes smooth, pliable, soft, and slightly tacky to the touch.
3. Remove the bread from the pan after baking. Place on rack and allow to cool for 1 hour before slicing.

Nutrition:

Calories: 65 Cal

Fat : 0 g

Carbohydrates: 13 g

Protein: 2 g

CHAPTER 9:

Sourdough Bread

5. Garlic and Herb Flatbread Sourdough

Preparation Time: 1 hour

Cooking Time: 25- 30 minutes

Servings: 12

Ingredients:

- Dough
- 1 cup sourdough starter, fed or unfed
- 3/4 cup warm water
- teaspoons instant yeast
- cups all-purpose flour
- 1 1/2 teaspoons salt
- tablespoons olive oil
- Topping
- 1/2 teaspoon dried thyme
- 1/2 teaspoon dried oregano
- 1/2 teaspoon dried marjoram
- 1 teaspoon garlic powder

- 1/4 teaspoon onion powder
- 1/4 teaspoon salt
- 1/4 teaspoon pepper
- 3 tablespoons olive oil

Directions:

1. Combine all the dough ingredients in the bowl of a stand mixer, and knead until smooth. Place in a lightly greased bowl and let rise for at least one hour. Punch down, then let rise again for at least one hour.
2. To prepare the topping, mix all ingredients except the olive oil in a small bowl.
3. Lightly grease a 9x13 baking pan or standard baking sheet, and pat and roll the dough into a long rectangle in the pan. Brush the olive oil over the dough, and sprinkle the herb and seasoning mixture over top. Cover and let rise for 15-20 minutes.
4. Preheat oven to 425F and bake for 25-30 minutes.

Nutrition:

Calories: 89 Cal

Fat: 3.7 g

Protein: 1.8 g

CHAPTER 10:

Sweet Bread

6. Brownie Bread

Preparation Time: 1 hour 15 minutes

Cooking Time: 50 minutes

Servings: 1 loaf

Ingredients:

- 1 egg
- 1 egg yolk
- 1 teaspoon Salt
- 1/2 cup boiling water
- 1/2 cup cocoa powder, unsweetened
- 1/2 cup warm water
- 1/2 teaspoon Active dry yeast
- tablespoon Vegetable oil
- teaspoon White sugar
- 2/3 cup white sugar
- cups bread flour

Directions:

1. Put the cocoa powder in a small bow. Pour boiling water and dissolve the cocoa powder.
2. Put the warm water, yeast and the 2 teaspoon White sugar in another bowl. Dissolve yeast and sugar. Let stand for about 10 minutes, or until the mix is creamy.
3. Place the cocoa mix, the yeast mix, the flour, the 2/3 cup white sugar, the salt, the vegetable, and the egg in the bread pan. Select basic bread cycle. Press start.

Nutrition:

Calories: 70 Cal

Fat   : 3 g

Carbohydrates: 10 g

Protein: 1 g

7. Black Forest Bread

Preparation Time: 2 hour 15 minutes

Cooking Time: 50 minutes

Servings: 1 loaf

Ingredients:

- 1 1/8 cups Warm water
- 1/3 cup Molasses
- 1 1/2 tablespoons Canola oil
- 1 1/2 cups Bread flour
- 1 cup Rye flour
- 1 cup Whole wheat flour
- 1 1/2 teaspoons Salt
- tablespoons Cocoa powder
- 1 1/2 tablespoons Caraway seeds
- teaspoons Active dry yeast

Directions:

1. Place all ingredients into your bread maker according to manufacture.
2. Select type to a light crust.
3. Press start.
4. Remembering to check while starting to knead.

5 If mixture is too dry add tablespoon warm water at a time.
6 If mixture is too wet add flour again a little at a time.
7 Mixture should go into a ball form, and just soft and slightly sticky to the finger touch. This goes for all types of bread when kneading.

Nutrition:

Calories: 240 Cal

Fat   : 4 g

Carbohydrates: 29 g

Protein: 22 g

CHAPTER 11:

Cheese Bread

8. Parmesan Tomato Basil Bread

Preparation Time: 5 Minutes

Cooking Time: 2 Hours

Servings: 10

Ingredients:

- Sun-dried tomatoes – ¼ cup, chopped
- Yeast – 2 tsp.
- Bread flour – 2 cups.
- Parmesan cheese – 1/3 cup, grated
- Dried basil – 2 tsp.
- Sugar – 1 tsp.
- Olive oil – 2 tbsp.
- Milk – ¼ cup.
- Water – ½ cup.
- Salt – 1 tsp.

Directions:

1. Add all ingredients except for sun-dried tomatoes into the bread machine pan.
2. Select the basic setting, then select medium crust and press start.
3. Add sun-dried tomatoes just before the final kneading cycle.
4. Once the loaf is done, remove the loaf pan from the machine.
5. Allow it to cool for 10 minutes
6. Slice and serve.

Nutrition:

Calories 183

Carbs 20.3g

Fat 6.8g

Protein 7.9g

9. Cheese Buttermilk Bread

Preparation Time: 5 Minutes

Cooking Time: 2 Hours

Servings: 10

Ingredients:

- Buttermilk – 1 1/8 cups
- Active dry yeast – 1 ½ tsp.
- Cheddar cheese – ¾ cup., shredded
- Sugar – 1 ½ tsp.
- Bread flour – 3 cups.
- Buttermilk – 1 1/8 cups.
- Salt – 1 1/2 tsp.

Directions:

1. Place all ingredients into the bread machine pan based on the bread machine manufacturer instructions.
2. Select basic bread setting, then select light/medium crust and start.
3. Once the loaf is done, remove the loaf pan from the machine.
4. Allow it to cool for 10 minutes.

5   Slice and serve.

Nutrition:

Calories 182

Carbs 30g

Fat 3.4g

Protein 6.8g

CHAPTER 12:

Dough Recipes

10. Cheddar Biscuits

Preparation Time: 10 minutes
Cooking Time: 25 minutes
Servings: 12

Ingredients:

- eggs
- ¼ cup unsalted butter, melted
- 1 ¼ cups, coconut milk
- ¼ tsp. salt
- ¼ tsp. baking soda
- ¼ tsp. garlic powder
- ½ cup finely shredded sharp cheddar cheese
- 1 Tbsp. fresh herb
- 2/3 cup coconut flour

Directions:

1. Preheat the oven to 350F. Grease a baking sheet.
2. Mix together the butter, eggs, milk, salt, baking soda, garlic powder, cheese, and herbs until well blended.
3. Add the coconut flour to the batter and mix until well blended. Let the batter sit then mix again.
4. Spoon about 2 tbsp. batter for each biscuit onto the greased baking sheet.
5. Bake for 25 minutes.
6. Serve warm.

Nutrition:

Calories: 125

Fat: 7g

Carb: 10g

Protein: 5g

CHAPTER 13:

Buns & Bread

11. Buns with Cottage Cheese

Preparation Time: 10 minutes

Cooking Time: 15 minutes

Servings: 8

Ingredients:

- eggs
- oz. Almond flour
- 1 oz. Erythritol
- 1/8 tsp. Stevia
- cinnamon and vanilla extract to taste Filling:
- ½ oz. Cottage cheese
- 1 egg
- cinnamon and vanilla extract to taste

Directions:

1 Prepare the filling by mixing its ingredients in a bowl.

2. Combine eggs with almond flour, blend until smooth. Add erythritol, stevia, and flavors to taste.
3. Spoon 1 tbsp. Dough into silicone cups. Spoon about 1 tsp. Filling on top, and bake at 365f for 15 minutes.

Nutrition:

Calories: 77

Fat: 5.2g

Carb: 6.7g

Protein: 5.8g

CHAPTER 14:

Bread machine recipes

12. Great Plum Bread

Preparation Time: 10 minutes

Cooking Time: 50 minutes

Servings: 8

Ingredients:

- 1 cup plums, pitted and chopped
- 1 and ½ cups coconut flour
- ¼ teaspoon baking soda
- ½ cup ghee, melted
- A pinch of salt
- 1 and ¼ cups swerve
- ½ teaspoon vanilla extract
- 1/3 cup coconut cream
- eggs, whisked

Directions:

1. Using a bowl, mix the flour with baking soda, salt, swerve, and the vanilla and stir.
2. Using a separate bowl, mix the plums with the remaining ingredients and stir.
3. Combine the 2 mixtures and stir the batter well.
4. Pour into 2 lined loaf pans and bake at temperature 350 degrees f for 50 minutes.
5. Cool the bread down, slice and serve them.

Nutrition:

Calories 199

Fat 8

Fiber 3

Carbs 6

Protein 4

13. Lime Bread

Preparation Time: 10 minutes
Cooking Time: 50 minutes
Servings: 8

Ingredients:

- 2/3 cup ghee, melted
- cups swerve
- eggs, whisked
- teaspoons baking powder
- 1 cup almond milk
- tablespoons lime zest, grated
- tablespoons lime juice
- cups coconut flour
- Cooking spray

Directions:

1. Using a bowl, mix the flour with lime zest, baking powder and the swerve and stir.
2. In a separate bowl, mix the lime juice with the rest of the ingredients except the cooking spray and stir well.

3. Combine the 2 mixtures, stir the batter well and pour into 2 loaf pans greased with cooking spray and bake at 350 degrees f for 50 minutes.
4. Cool the bread down, slice and serve.

Nutrition:

Calories 203

Fat 7

Fiber 3

Carbs 4

Protein 6

CHAPTER 15:

Nut and Seed Bread

14. Flax and Sunflower Seed Bread

Preparation Time: 5 Minutes

Cooking Time: 25 Minutes

Servings: 8

Ingredients:

- 1 1/3 cups water
- Two tablespoons butter softened
- Three tablespoons honey
- 2/3 cups of bread flour
- One teaspoon salt
- One teaspoon active dry yeast
- 1/2 cup flax seeds
- 1/2 cup sunflower seeds

Directions:

1. With the manufacturer's suggested order, add all the ingredients (apart from sunflower seeds) to the bread machine's pan.

2. The select basic white cycle, then press start.
3. Just in the knead cycle that your machine signals alert sounds, add the sunflower seeds.

Nutrition:

Calories: 140 calories;

Sodium: 169

Total Carbohydrate: 22.7

Cholesterol: 4

Protein: 4.2

Total Fat: 4.2

15. Honey and Flaxseed Bread

Preparation Time: 5 Minutes

Cooking Time: 25 Minutes

Servings: 8

Ingredients:

- 1 1/8 cups water
- 1 1/2 tablespoons flaxseed oil
- Three tablespoons honey
- 1/2 tablespoon liquid lecithin
- cups whole wheat flour
- 1/2 cup flax seed
- Two tablespoons bread flour
- Three tablespoons whey powder
- 1 1/2 teaspoons sea salt
- Two teaspoons active dry yeast

Directions:

1. In the bread machine pan, put in all of the ingredients following the order recommended by the manufacturer.

2   Choose the Wheat cycle on the machine and press the Start button to run the machine.

Nutrition:

Calories: 174 calories;

Protein: 7.1

Total Fat: 4.9

Sodium: 242

Total Carbohydrate: 30.8

Cholesterol: 1

CHAPTER 16:

Vegetable Bread

16. Banana-Lemon Loaf

Preparation Time: 15 minutes

Cooking Time: 1.5 hours

Serving Size: 1 ounce (28.3g)

Ingredients:

- 2 cups all-purpose flour
- 1 cup bananas, very ripe and mashed
- 1 cup walnuts, chopped
- 1 cup of sugar
- One tablespoon baking powder
- One teaspoon lemon peel, grated
- ½ teaspoon salt
- Two eggs
- ½ cup of vegetable oil
- Two tablespoons lemon juice

Direction:

1. Put all ingredients into a pan in this order: bananas, wet ingredients, and then dry ingredients.
2. Press the "Quick" or "Cake" setting of your bread machine.
3. Allow the cycles to be completed.
4. Take out the pan from the machine. The cooldown for 10 minutes before slicing the bread enjoy.

Nutrition:

Calories: 120 | Carbohydrates: 15g

Fat: 6g | Protein: 2g

17. Orange Date Bread

Preparation Time: 20 minutes

Cooking Time: 1.5 hours

Serving Size: 1 ounce (28.3g)

Ingredients:

- 2 cups all-purpose flour
- 1 cup dates, chopped
- ¾ cup of sugar
- ½ cup walnuts, chopped
- Two tablespoons orange rind, grated
- 1 ½ teaspoons baking powder
- One teaspoon baking soda
- ½ cup of orange juice
- ½ cup of water
- One tablespoon vegetable oil
- One teaspoon vanilla extract

Direction:

1. Put the wet ingredients then the dry ingredients into the bread pan.
2. Press the "Quick" or "Cake" mode of the bread machine.

3. Allow all cycles to be finished.
4. Remove the pan from the machine, but keep the bread in the pan for 10 minutes more.
5. Take out the bread from the pan, and let it cool down completely before slicing.

Nutrition:

Calories: 80 | Carbohydrates: 14g

Fat: 2g | Protein: 1g

CHAPTER 17:

Basic Bread

18. Gluten-Free Bread

Preparation Time: 4 hours 50 minutes
Cooking Time: 50 minutes (20+30 minutes)
Servings: 1 loaf

Ingredients:

- 2 cups rice flour, Potato starch
- 1 1/2 cup Tapioca flour
- 1/2 cup Xanthan gum
- 2 1/2 teaspoons 2/3 cup powdered milk or 1/2 non-dairy substitute
- 1 1/2 teaspoons salt
- 1 1/2 teaspoons egg substitute (optional)
- Three tablespoons Sugar
- 1 2/3 cups lukewarm water
- 1 1/2 tablespoons dry yeast, granules
- Four tablespoons butter, melted or margarine

- One teaspoon Vinegar
- Three eggs, room temperature

Directions:
1. Add yeast to the bread pan.
2. Add all the flours, xanthan/ gum, milk powder, salt, and sugar.
3. Beat the eggs, and mix with water, butter, and vinegar.
4. Choose white bread setting at medium or use a 3-4-hour set.

Nutrition:

Calories: 126 Cal

Fat: 2 g

Carbohydrates: 29 g

Protein: 3 g

CHAPTER 18:

Pleasure Bread

19. Crisp White Bread

Preparation Time: 2 hours and 30 minutes

Cooking Time: 1 hour and 30 minutes.

Servings: 1-pound loaf / 10 slices

Ingredients:

- ¾ cup lukewarm water (80 degrees F)
- One tablespoon butter, melted
- One tablespoon white sugar
- ¾ teaspoon sea salt
- Two tablespoons of milk powder
- 2 cups wheat flour
- ¾ teaspoon active dry yeast

Direction:

1. Prepare all of the ingredients for your bread and measuring means (a cup, a spoon, kitchen scales).

2. Carefully measure the ingredients into the pan.
3. Put all the ingredients into a bread bucket in the right order, following the manual for your bread machine.
4. Close the cover. Select your bread machine program to BASIC / WHITE BREAD and choose the crust colour to MEDIUM.
5. Press START. Wait until the program completes.
6. When done, take the bucket out and let it cool for 5-10 minutes.
7. Shake the loaf from the pan and let cool for 30 minutes on a cooling rack.
8. Slice and serve.

Nutrition:

Calories 113; Total Fat 1.4g; Saturated Fat 0.8g; Cholesterol 3g; Sodium 158mg; Total Carbohydrate 21.6g; Dietary Fiber 0.7g; Total Sugars 2.1g; Protein 3.3g, Vitamin D 1mcg, Calcium 24mg, Iron 1mg, Potassium 33mg

CHAPTER 19:

Cakes and Quick Bread

20. Honey Pound Cake

Preparation Time: 5 minutes

Cooking Time: 2 hours 50 minutes

Servings: 12 - 16

Ingredients:

- 1 cup butter, unsalted
- 1/4 cup honey
- Two tablespoons whole milk
- Four eggs, beaten
- 1 cup of sugar
- 2 cups flour

Direction:

1. Bring the butter to room temperature and cut into 1/2-inch cubes.
2. Add all ingredients to the bread machine in the order listed (butter, honey, milk, eggs, sugar, and flour).

3. Press Sweetbread setting follow by light crust colour, then press Start. Take out the cake on the bread pan using a rubber spatula as soon as it's finished. Cool on a rack and serve with your favorite fruit.

Nutrition:

Calories: 117, Sodium: 183 mg, Dietary Fiber: 0.3 g, Fat: 6.9 g, Carbs: 12.3 g, Protein: 1.9 g.

CHAPTER 20:

Meat Bread

21. French Ham Bread

Preparation Time: 30-45 minutes
Cooking Time: 2 hours
Servings: 8

Ingredients:

- 3 1/3 cups wheat flour
- 1 cup ham
- ½ cup of milk powder
- 1 ½ tablespoons sugar
- One teaspoon yeast, fresh
- One teaspoon salt
- One teaspoon dried basil
- 1 1/3 cups water
- Two tablespoons olive oil

Directions:
1. Cut ham into cubes of 0.5-1 cm (approximately ¼ inch).
2. Put all ingredients in the bread maker from the following order: water, olive oil, salt, sugar, flour, milk powder, ham, and yeast.
3. Put all the ingredients according to the instructions in your bread maker.
4. Basil put in a dispenser or fill it later, at the signal in the container.
5. Turn on the bread maker.
6. After the end of the baking cycle, leave the bread container
7. In the bread maker to keep warm for 1 hour.
8. Then your delicious bread is ready!

Nutrition:

Calories 287

Total Fat 5.5g

Saturated Fat 1.1g

Cholesterol 11g

Sodium 557mg

Total Carbohydrate 47.2g

Dietary Fiber 1.7g

Total Sugars 6.4g

Protein 11.4g

CHAPTER 21:

Multi-Grain Bread

22. French Crusty Loaf Bread

Preparation Time: 2 hours

Cooking Time: 1 hour

Servings: 1 loaf

Ingredients:

- 16 slice bread (2 pounds)
- 2 cups + 2 tablespoons water, lukewarm between 80 and 90 degrees F
- Four teaspoons sugar
- Two teaspoons table salt
- 6 1/2 cups white bread flour
- Two teaspoons bread machine yeast
- 12 slice bread (1 ½ pound)
- 1 1/2 cups + 1 tablespoon water, lukewarm between 80 and 90 degrees F
- Three teaspoons sugar
- 1 1/2 teaspoons table salt

- 4 3/4 cups white bread flour
- 1 1/2 teaspoons bread machine yeast

Directions:

1. Choose the size of loaf you would like to make and measure your ingredients.
2. Put the ingredients to the bread pan in the order list above.
3. Place the pan in the machine and close the lid.
4. Switch on the bread maker. Select the French setting, then the loaf size, and finally, the crust colour. Start the cycle.
5. When the process is finished and the bread is baked, remove the pan from the machine. Use a potholder as the handle. Rest for a few minutes.
6. Take out the bread from the pan and let it cool on a wire rack for at least 10 minutes before slicing.

Nutrition:

Calories 186, Fat 1.2 g, carbs 31.4 g, sodium 126 mg, protein 5.7 g

CHAPTER 22:

Holiday Bread

23. Pumpkin Bread

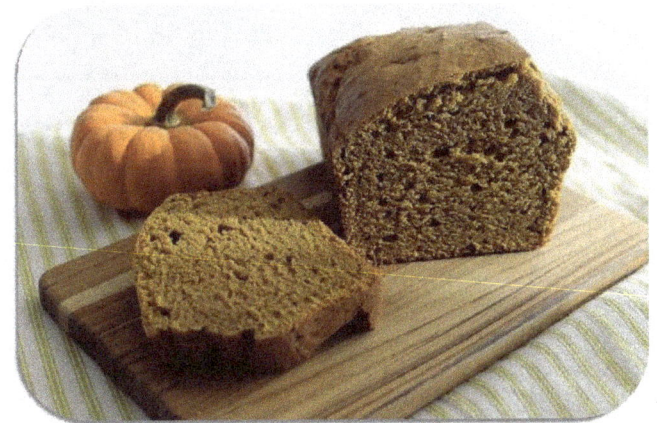

Preparation Time: 5 minutes

Cooking Time: 1 hour

Servings: 14

Ingredients:

- ½ cup plus 2 tablespoons warm water
- ½ cup canned pumpkin puree
- ¼ cup butter, softened
- ¼ cup non-fat dry milk powder

- 2¾ cups bread flour
- ¼ cup brown sugar
- ¾ teaspoon salt
- 1 teaspoon ground cinnamon
- ½ teaspoon ground ginger
- 1/8 teaspoon ground nutmeg
- 2¼ teaspoons active dry yeast

Directions:
1. Place all ingredients in the baking pan of the bread machine in the order recommended by the manufacturer.
2. Place the baking pan in the bread machine and close the lid.
3. Select Basic setting.
4. Press the start button.
5. Carefully, remove the baking pan from the machine and then invert the bread loaf onto a wire rack to cool completely before slicing.
6. With a sharp knife, cut bread loaf into desired-sized slices and serve.

Nutrition:
Calories 134, Total Fat 3.6 g, Saturated Fat 2.1 g, Cholesterol 9 mg, Sodium 149 mg, Total Carbs 22.4 g, Fiber 1.1 g, Sugar 2.9 g, Protein 2.9 g

CHAPTER 23:

Keto Bread Recipes

24. Simple Milk Bread

Preparation Time: 3 minutes

Cooking Time: 3 minutes

Servings: 8

Ingredients:

- cups almond flour
- tbsp. inulin
- 1 tbsp. whole milk
- ½ tsp. salt
- tsp. active yeast
- 1 ¼ cups warm water
- 1 tbsp. olive oil

Directions:

1. Use a small mixing bowl to combine all dry Ingredients, except for the yeast.
2. In the bread machine pan add all wet Ingredients.

3. Add all of your dry Ingredients, from the small mixing bowl, in the bread machine pan. Top with the yeast.
4. Set the bread machine to the basic bread setting.
5. When the bread is done, remove bread machine pan from the bread machine.
6. Let cool slightly before transferring to a cooling rack.
7. The bread can be stored for up to 5 days on the counter and for up to 3 months in the freezer.

Nutrition: carbohydrates 4 g fats 7 g protein 3 g calories 85 Fiber 1.5 g

25. Toast Bread

Preparation Time: 3 ½ hours
Cooking Time: 3 ½ hours
Servings: 8

Ingredients:

- 1 ½ teaspoons yeast
- cups almond flour
- tablespoons sugar
- 1 teaspoon salt
- 1 ½ tablespoon butter
- 1 cup water

Directions:

1. Pour water into the bowl; add salt, sugar, soft butter, flour, and yeast.
2. I add dried tomatoes and paprika.
3. Put it on the basic program.
4. The crust can be light or medium.

Nutrition: carbohydrates 5 g fats 2.7 g protein 5.2 g calories 203 fiber 1 g

26. Walnut Bread

Preparation Time: 4 hours
Cooking Time: 4 hours
Servings: 10

Ingredients:

- cups almond flour
- ½ cup water
- ½ cup milk
- eggs
- ½ cup walnuts
- 1 tablespoon vegetable oil
- 1 tablespoon sugar
- 1 teaspoon salt
- 1 teaspoon yeast

Directions

1. All products must be room temperature.
2. Pour water, milk, and vegetable oil into the bucket and add in the eggs.
3. Now pour in the sifted almond flour. In the process of kneading bread, you may need a little more or less flour – it depends on its moisture.

4. Pour in salt, sugar, and yeast. If it is hot in the kitchen (especially in summer), pour all three Ingredients into the different ends of the bucket so that the dough does not have time for peroxide.
5. Now the first kneading dough begins, which lasts 15 minutes. In the process, we monitor the state of the ball. It should be soft, but at the same time, keep its shape and not spread. If the ball does not want to be collected, add a little flour, since the moisture of this product is different for everyone. If the bucket is clean and all the flour is incorporated into the dough, then everything is done right. If the dough is still lumpy and even crumbles, you need to add a little more liquid.
6. Close the lid and then prepare the nuts. They need to be sorted and lightly fried in a dry frying pan; the pieces of nuts will be crispy. Then let them cool and cut with a knife to the desired size. When the bread maker signals, pour in the nuts and wait until the spatula mixes them into the dough.
7. Remove the bucket and take out the walnut bread. Completely cool it on a grill so that the bottom does not get wet.

Nutrition: carbohydrates 4 g fats 6.7 g protein 8.3 g calories 257 fiber 1.3 g

CHAPTER 24:

International Bread

27. German Pumpernickel Bread

Preparation Time: 2 hours

Cooking Time: 1 hour and 10 minutes.

Servings: 1 loaf

Ingredients:

- 1 1/2 tablespoon vegetable oil
- 1 1/8 cups warm water
- Three tablespoons cocoa
- 1/3 cup molasses
- 1 ½ teaspoons salt
- One tablespoon caraway seeds
- 1 cup rye flour
- 1 ½ cups of bread flour
- 1 ½ tablespoon wheat gluten
- 1 cup whole wheat flour
- 2 ½ teaspoons bread machine yeast

Directions:

1. Put everything in your bread machine.
2. Select the primary cycle.
3. Hit the start button.
4. Transfer bread to a rack for cooling once done.

Nutrition:

Calories 119, Carbohydrates 22.4 g, Total Fat 2.3 g, Cholesterol 0mg, Protein 3 g, Sodium 295 mg

CHAPTER 25:

Fruit and Vegetable Bread

28. Banana Bread

Preparation Time: 1 hour 40 minutes

Cooking Time: 40- 45 minutes

Servings: 1 loaf

Ingredients:

- One teaspoon Baking powder
- 1/2 teaspoon Baking soda
- Two bananas, peeled and halved lengthwise
- 2 cups all-purpose flour
- Two eggs
- Three tablespoon Vegetable oil
- 3/4 cup white sugar

Directions:

1. Put all the ingredients in the bread pan—select dough setting. Start and mix for about 3-5 minutes.

2. After 3-5 minutes, press stop. Do not continue to mix. Smooth out the top of the dough

3. Using the spatula and then select bake, start and bake for about 50 minutes. After 50 minutes, insert a toothpick into the top center to test doneness.

4. Test the loaf again. When the bread is completely baked, remove the pan from the machine and let the bread remain in the pan for10 minutes. Remove bread and cool in a wire rack.

Nutrition:

Calories: 310 calories

Total Carbohydrate: 40 g

Fat: 13 g

Protein: 3 g

29. Orange and Walnut Bread

Preparation Time: 2 hours 50 minutes

Cooking Time: 45 minutes

Servings: 10- 15

Ingredients:

- One egg white
- One tablespoon water
- ½ cup warm whey
- One tablespoons yeast
- Four tablespoons sugar
- Two oranges, crushed
- 4 cups flour
- One teaspoon salt
- One and ½ tablespoon salt
- Three teaspoons orange peel
- 1/3 teaspoon vanilla
- Three tablespoons walnut and almonds, crushed
- Crushed pepper, salt, cheese for garnish

Directions:

1. Put all of the ingredients in your Bread Machine (except egg white, one tablespoon water, and crushed pepper/ cheese).

2. Set the program to the "Dough" cycle and let the cycle run.
3. Remove the dough (using lightly floured hands) and carefully place it on a floured surface.
4. Cover with a light film/cling paper and let the dough rise for 10 minutes.
5. Divide the dough into thirds after it has risen
6. Place on a light flour surface, roll each portion into 14x10 inch sized rectangles
7. Use a sharp knife to cut carefully cut the dough into strips of ½ inch width
8. Pick 2-3 strips and twist them multiple times, making sure to press the ends together
9. Preheat your oven to 400 degrees F
10. Take a bowl and stir egg white, water, and brush onto the breadsticks
11. Sprinkle salt, pepper/ cheese
12. Bake for 10-12 minutes until golden brown
13. Remove from the baking sheet, then transfer to a cooling rack. Serve and enjoy!

Nutrition:

Calories: 437 calories;

Total Carbohydrate: 82 g

Total Fat: 7 g

Protein: 12 g, Sugar: 34 g, Fiber: 1 g

CHAPTER 26:

White Bread

30. Basic White Bread

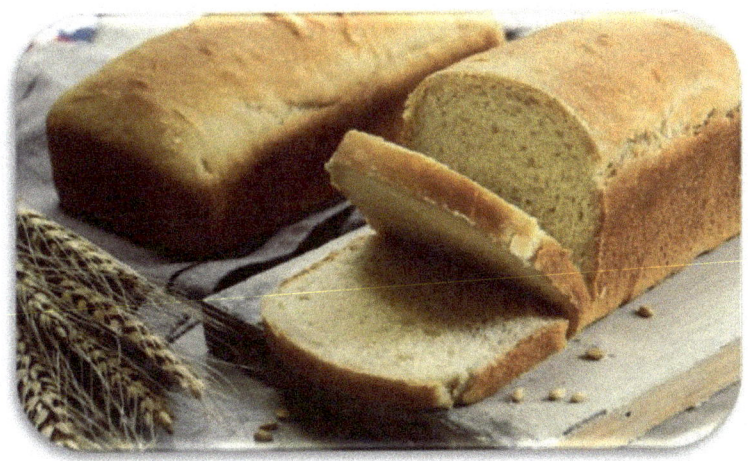

Preparation Time: 5 minutes

Cooking Time: 3 hours

Servings: 16

Ingredients:

- 1 cup warm water (about 110°F/45°C)
- 2 Tablespoon sugar
- 2¼ teaspoon (.25-ounce package) bread machine yeast

- ¼ cup rice bran oil
- 3 cups bread flour
- 1 teaspoon salt

Directions:

1. Add each ingredient to the bread machine in the order and at the temperature recommended by your bread machine manufacturer.
2. Close the lid, select the basic or white bread, low crust setting on your bread machine, and press start.
3. When the bread machine has finished baking, remove the bread and put it on a cooling rack.

Nutrition:

Carbs: 18 g

Fat: 1 g

Protein: 3 g

Calories: 95

CHAPTER 27:

Special Bread Recipes

31. Gluten-Free Simple Sandwich Bread

Preparation Time: 5 Minutes

Cooking Time: 60 Minutes

Servings: 12

Ingredients:

- 1 1/2 cups sorghum flour
- 1 cup tapioca starch or potato starch
- 1/3 cup gluten-free millet flour or gluten-free oat flour
- Two teaspoons xanthan gum
- 1 1/4 teaspoons fine sea salt
- 2 1/2 teaspoons gluten-free yeast for bread machines
- 1 1/4 cups warm water
- Three tablespoons extra virgin olive oil
- One tablespoon honey or raw agave nectar
- 1/2 teaspoon mild rice vinegar or lemon juice
- Two organic free-range eggs, beaten

Directions:

1. Blend the dry ingredients except for the yeast and set aside.
2. Add the liquid ingredients to the bread maker pan first, then gently pour the mixed dry ingredients on top of the liquid.
3. Make a well in the center part of the dry ingredients and add the yeast.
4. Set for Rapid 1 hour 20 minutes, medium crust color, and press Start.
5. In the end, put it on a cooling rack for 15 minutes before slicing to serve.

Nutrition:

Calories: 137

Sodium: 85 mg

Dietary Fiber: 2.7 g

Fat: 4.6 g

Carbs: 22.1 g

Protein: 2.4 g

32. Grain-Free Chia Bread

Preparation Time: 5 Minutes

Cooking Time: 3 Hours

Servings: 12

Ingredients:

- 1 cup of warm water
- Three large organic eggs, room temperature
- 1/4 cup olive oil
- One tablespoon apple cider vinegar
- 1 cup gluten-free chia seeds, ground to flour
- 1 cup almond meal flour
- 1/2 cup potato starch
- 1/4 cup coconut flour
- 3/4 cup millet flour
- One tablespoon xanthan gum
- 1 1/2 teaspoons salt
- Two tablespoons sugar
- Three tablespoons nonfat dry milk
- Six teaspoons instant yeast

Directions:

1. Whisk wet ingredients together and place it in the bread maker pan.
2. Whisk dry ingredients, except yeast, together, and add on top of wet ingredients.
3. Make a well in the dry ingredients and add yeast.
4. Select the Whole Wheat cycle, light crust color, and press Start.
5. Allow cooling completely before serving.

Nutrition:

Calories: 375

Sodium: 462 mg

Dietary Fiber: 22.3 g

Fat: 18.3 g

Carbs: 42 g

Protein: 12.2 g

CHAPTER 28:

Rolls and Pizza

33. Sweet Potato Rolls

Preparation Time: 25 Minutes

Cooking Time: 40 Minutes

Servings: 8

Ingredients:

- Two meshed medium sweet potatoes
- 1 cup milk
- 3.2 tablespoons melted butter
- 1 large beaten egg
- 4 cups all-purpose flour
- 4 tablespoons sugar
- 1 teaspoon salt
- 2.5 teaspoons active dry yeast

Directions:

1. Peel potatoes and cut in cubes

2. Boil salted water
3. Add potato to water and reduce the heat. Cover the pan and cook for about 22 minutes
4. Drain and mash
5. Cool and measure 1 cup
6. Add Ingredients to the bread machine according to manufacturer's recommendations
7. Use the basic dough cycle
8. When it finishes, tear pieces to make balls, place in a baking pan
9. Cover rolls through a cloth and let rise for about 40 minutes
10. Preheat oven to 370 F
11. Bake until nicely browned
12. Brush the tops with melted or softened butter

Nutrition:

Carbs – 28 G

Fat – 3 G

Protein – 6 G

Calories – 160

CHAPTER 29:

Italian Styled

34. Fruit Bread

Preparation Time: 3 hours

Cooking Time: 0

Servings: 8

Ingredients:

- 1 egg
- 1 cup milk
- tablespoons rum
- ¼ cup butter
- ¼ cup brown sugar
- cups almond flour
- 1 tablespoon instant yeast
- 1 teaspoon salt
- Fruits:
- ¼ cups dried apricots, coarsely chopped
- ¼ cups prunes, coarsely chopped

- ¼ cups candied cherry, pitted
- ½ cups seedless raisins
- ¼ cup almonds, chopped

Directions:

1. Put all of the ingredients to your bread machine, carefully following the instructions of the manufacturer (except fruits).
2. Set the program of your bread machine to basic/sweet and set crust type to light or medium.
3. Press starts.
4. Once the machine beeps, add fruits.
5. Wait until the cycle completes.
6. Once the loaf is ready, take the bucket out and let the loaf cool for 5 minutes.
7. Gently shake the bucket to remove loaf.
8. Move it to a cooling rack, slice and serve.
9. Enjoy!

Nutrition:

Carbohydrates 5 g

Fats 10.9 g

Protein 10.8 g

Calories 441

35. Marzipan Cherry Bread

Preparation Time: 3 hours

Cooking Time: 0

Servings: 8

Ingredients:

- 1 egg
- ¾ cup milk
- 1 tablespoon almond liqueur
- tablespoons orange juice
- ½ cup ground almonds
- ¼ cup butter
- 1/3 cup sugar
- cups almond flour
- 1 tablespoon instant yeast
- 1 teaspoon salt
- ½ cup marzipan
- ½ cup dried cherries, pitted

Directions:

1. Put all of the ingredients to your bread machine, carefully following the instructions of the manufacturer (except marzipan and cherry).

2. Set the program of your bread machine to basic/sweet and set crust type to light or medium.
3. Press starts.
4. Once the machine beeps, add marzipan and cherry.
5. Wait until the cycle completes.
6. Once the loaf is ready, take the bucket out and let the loaf cool for 5 minutes.
7. Gently shake the bucket to remove loaf.
8. Move it to a cooling rack, slice and serve.
9. Enjoy!

Nutrition:

Carbohydrates 4.2 g

Fats 16.4 g

Protein 12.2 g

Calories 511

36. Ginger Prune Bread

Preparation Time: 3 hours

Cooking Time: 0

Servings: 8

Ingredients:

- eggs
- 1 cup milk
- ¼ cup butter
- ¼ cup sugar
- cups almond flour
- 1 tablespoon instant yeast
- 1 teaspoon salt
- 1 cup prunes, coarsely chopped
- 1 tablespoon fresh ginger, grated

Directions:

1. Put all of the ingredients to your bread machine, carefully following the instructions of the manufacturer (except ginger and prunes).
2. Set the program of your bread machine to basic/sweet and set crust type to light or medium.
3. Press starts.

4. Once the machine beeps, add ginger and prunes.
5. Wait until the cycle completes.
6. Once the loaf is ready, take the bucket out and let the loaf cool for 5 minutes.
7. Gently shake the bucket to remove loaf.
8. Move it to a cooling rack, slice and serve.
9. Enjoy!

Nutrition:

Carbohydrates 4 g

Fats 8.3 g

Protein 10.1 g

Calories 387

CHAPTER 30:

Famous Bread Recipes

37. Bread Machine Glazed Yeast Doughnuts

Preparation Time: 25 Minutes

Cooking Time: 20 Minutes

Servings: 20

Ingredients:

- 1/2 cup evaporated milk
- 1/2 cup water
- 2 tbsp. butter
- One large egg, beaten
- 1/3 cup sugar
- 3 cups all-purpose flour
- 1 tsp. salt
- 2 tsp. active dry yeast
- Oil for deep-frying

For the Chocolate Glaze

- 2 tbsp. butter

- 2 tbsp. cocoa
- 3 tbsp. hot water
- 1 1/2 cups powdered sugar
- 1/2 tsp. vanilla extract

Directions:
1. Add all the ingredients to the bread machine.
2. During the kneading cycle, you should cover the pan with plastic wrap and then transfer it to the refrigerator. (You may also transfer the mixture to a lightly greased bowl). Refrigerate overnight.
3. Remove the dough to a lightly floured surface and roll to about 1/2-inch thick.
4. Cut out into doughnut shapes or form strips into knots or cruller shapes. Do not forget to cover and let rise for about 1 hour.
5. Fry in oil at 360 F until light and brown. Now, glaze with the use of chocolate icing or use your favorite icing.
6. Chocolate or Vanilla Glaze
7. Melt butter in a small saucepan over low heat; add cocoa and water. Stir constantly until the mixture is thick.
8. Remove from heat, then gradually add powdered sugar and vanilla; beat with a whisk until smooth.
9. Add additional hot water, 1/2 teaspoon at a time, until drizzling constancy.

10. For the vanilla glaze, omit cocoa and add 1 1/2 teaspoons vanilla.

Nutrition:

Calories: 130 calories;

Total Carbohydrate: 18 g

Total Fat: 7 g

Protein: 1 g

38. Bread Machine Kalamata Olive Bread

Preparation Time: 10 Minutes

Cooking Time: 2 Hours

Servings: 10

Ingredients:

- 1/2 cup brine from olives
- 1 cup of warm water
- 2 tbsp. olive oil
- 3 cups bread flour
- 1 2/3 cups whole-wheat flour
- 1 1/2 tsp. salt
- 2 tsp. sugar
- 1 1/2 tsp. dried basil
- 2 tsp. active dry yeast
- 1/2 to 2/3 cup of finely chopped olives

Directions:

1. Put the olive brine in a 2-cup measure; add warm water to make 1 1/2 cups volume.
2. Place all ingredients, excluding the olives, in the bread machine according to your manufacturer's preferred order.
3. Choose the basic or wheat setting on your bread machine.

4. Add olives at the beep, indicating time to add mix-in ingredients.
5. When your loaf is finished baking, slice it and enjoy it by itself, with butter or olive oil.

Nutrition:

Calories: 130 calories;

Total Carbohydrate: 18 g

Total Fat: 7 g

Protein: 1 g

39. Dark Pumpernickel Bread

Preparation Time: 15 Minutes

Cooking Time: 2 Hours

Servings: 16

Ingredients:

- 1 1/3 cups strong coffee
- 1/4 cup vegetable oil
- 1/4 cup molasses
- 1 cup whole wheat flour
- 1 cup rye flour
- 2 cups bread flour
- 2 1/2 tsp. caraway seeds
- 2 tbsp. unsweetened cocoa
- 1 1/2 tbsp. brown sugar
- 1 tsp. salt
- 2 1/2 tsp. active dry yeast

Directions:

1. Fill bread machine and bake according to the bread machine manufacturer's recommendations.
2. To make a free-form loaf, use the dough cycle. Remove the dough and shape on a parchment-paper-lined baking sheet.

3. Cover the bread with a towel and allow it to rise for about 45 minutes to 1 hour in a draft-free place.
4. Bake in a warmed oven for around 25 to 35 minutes. The loaf should sound hollow when tapped on the bottom.

Nutrition:

Calories: 130 calories;

Total Carbohydrate: 18 g

Total Fat: 7 g

Protein: 1 g

40. Bread Machine Hamburger Buns

Preparation Time: 25 Minutes

Cooking Time: 18 Minutes

Servings: 8

Ingredients:

- 1 1/3 cups water
- 2 tbsp. nonfat milk powder
- 4 cups all-purpose flour
- 2 tbsp. shortening
- 3 tbsp. sugar
- 2 tsp. salt
- 2 1/2 tsp. active dry yeast
- Cornmeal
- One egg white (beaten with 1 tbsp. of water)
- Sesame seeds for topping

Directions:

1. Add the water and nonfat milk powder to the bread machine, followed by the flour. Add the shortening followed by the sugar, salt, and yeast. Set to the dough cycle.
2. When the bread machine finishes, turn the dough out onto a floured board and punch it down. Knead 4 or 5 times.

3. Cover the dough with a clean towel besides rest for about 30 minutes in a warm, dry place.
4. Lightly grease a large baking sheet; sprinkle with cornmeal. Alternatively, mark the baking sheet with parchment paper and sprinkle with cornmeal.
5. Pat the dough into a circle and cut into eight even wedges. Form each wedge into a ball, and then flatten each one into a smooth and reasonably even circle, slightly bigger than a burger.
6. Assemble the dough pieces on the baking sheet about 2 inches apart and rest for around 20 minutes.
7. Preheat the oven.
8. Brush the buns lightly utilizing the egg wash (a mixture of egg and water). If chosen, sprinkle with sesame seeds.
9. Bake the buns for around 18 minutes or until the buns are nicely browned.
10. Let cool before serving.

Nutrition:

Calories: 130 calories;

Total Carbohydrate: 18 g

Total Fat: 7 g

Protein: 3 g

Conclusion

This book has presented you with some of the easiest and delicious bread recipes you can find.

These loaves of bread are made using the everyday ingredients you can find locally, so there's no need to order anything or go to any specialty stores for any of them. With these pieces of bread, you can enjoy the same meals you used to enjoy but stay on track with your diet as much as you want.

Moreover, we have learned that the bread machine is a vital tool to have in our kitchen. It is not that hard to put into use. All you need to learn is how it functions and what its features are. You also need to use it more often to learn the dos and don'ts of using the machine.

The bread machine comes with instructions that you must learn from the manual to use it the right way. There is a certain way of loading the ingredients that must be followed, and the instructions vary according to the make and the model. So, when you first get a machine, sit down and learn the manual from start to finish; this allows you to put it to good use and get better results. The manual will tell you exactly what to put in it, as well as the correct settings to use, according to the different ingredients and the type of bread you want to make.

Having a bread machine in your kitchen makes life easy. Whether you are a professional baker or a home cook, this appliance will help you get the best bread texture and flavors with minimum effort. Bread making is an art, and it takes extra care and special technique to deal with a specific type of flour and bread machine that enables you to do so even when you are not a professional. In this book, we have discussed all bread machines and how we can put them to good use. Basic information about flour and yeast is also discussed to give all the beginners an idea of how to deal with the major ingredients of bread and what variety to use to get a particular type of bread. And finally, some delicious bread recipes were shared so that you can try them at home!

Conversion Tables

Measuring Equivalent Chart

3 teaspoons	1 tablespoon
2 tablespoons	1 ounce
4 tablespoons	¼ cup
8 tablespoons	½ cup
16 tablespoons	1 cup
2 cups	1 pint
4 cups	1 quart
4 quarts	1 gallon

Type	Imperial	Imperial	Metric
Weight	1 dry ounce		28g
	1 pound	16 dry ounces	0.45 kg
Volume	1 teaspoon		5 ml
	1 dessert spoon	2 teaspoons	10 ml
	1 tablespoon	3 teaspoons	15 ml
	1 Australian tablespoon	4 teaspoons	20 ml
	1 fluid ounce	2 tablespoons	30 ml
	1 cup	16 tablespoons	240 ml
	1 cup	8 fluid ounces	240 ml
	1 pint	2 cups	470 ml
	1 quart	2 pints	0.95 l
	1 gallon	4 quarts	3.8 l
Length	1 inch		2.54 cm

* Numbers are rounded to the closest equivalent

Gluten-Free – Conversion Tables

All-Purpose Flour	Rice Flour	Potato Starch	Tapioca	Xanthan Gum
½ cup	1/3 cup	2 tablespoons	1 tablespoon	¼ teaspoon
1 cup	½ cup	3 tablespoons	1 tablespoon	½ teaspoon
¼ cup	¾ cup	1/3 cup	3 tablespoons	2/3 teaspoon
1 ½ cup	1 cup	5 tablespoons	3 tablespoons	2/3 teaspoon
1 ¾ cup	1 ¼ cup	5 tablespoons	3 tablespoons	1 teaspoon
2 cups	1 ½ cup	1/3 cup	1/3 cup	1 teaspoon
2 ½ cups	1 ½ cup	½ cup	¼ cup	1 1/8 teaspoon
2 2/3 cups	2 cups	½ cup	¼ cup	1 ¼ teaspoon
3 cups	2 cups	2/3 cup	1/3 cup	1 ½ cup

Flour: Quantity and Weight

Flour Amount
1 cup = 140 grams
3/4 cup = 105 grams
1/2 cup = 70 grams
1/4 cup = 35 grams

Sugar: Quantity and Weight

Sugar
1 cup = 200 grams
3/4 cup = 150 grams
2/3 cup = 135 grams
1/2 cup = 100 grams
1/3 cup = 70 grams
1/4 cup = 50 grams

Powdered Sugar
1 cup = 160 grams
3/4 cup = 120 grams
1/2 cup = 80 grams
1/4 cup = 40 grams

Cream: Quantity and Weight

Cream Amount
1 cup = 250 ml = 235 grams
3/4 cup = 188 ml = 175 grams
1/2 cup = 125 ml = 115 grams
1/4 cup = 63 ml = 60 grams
1 tablespoon = 15 ml = 15 grams

Butter: Quantity and Weight

Butter Amount
1 cup = 8 ounces = 2 sticks = 16 tablespoons = 230 grams
1/2 cup = 4 ounces = 1 stick = 8 tablespoons = 115 grams
¼ cup = 2 ounces = ½ stick = 4 tablespoons = 58 grams

Oven Temperature Equivalent Chart

Fahrenheit (°F)	Celsius (°C)	Gas Mark
220	100	
225	110	1/4
250	120	1/2
275	140	1
300	150	2
325	160	3
350	180	4
375	190	5
400	200	6
425	220	7
450	230	8
475	250	9
500	260	

* Celsius (°C) = T (°F)-32] * 5/9

** Fahrenheit (°F) = T (°C) * 9/5 + 32

*** Numbers are rounded to the closest equivalent

CPSIA information can be obtained
at www.ICGtesting.com
Printed in the USA
LVHW080142230521
688251LV00002B/91